TABLE OF CONTENT

CHAPTER 1: THE BEGINNING

- **My Struggles with Weight**
  - o Early life and weight issues
  - o Emotional and psychological impacts
- **Societal Perceptions and Labels**
  - o How society views weight
  - o Personal experiences with being called "fat"
- **Decision to Change**
  - o The turning point
  - o Setting the stage for transformation

CHAPTER 2: UNDERSTANDING WEIGHT LOSS

- **The Science of Weight Loss**
    - o Basics of metabolism and calorie balance
    - o Importance of nutrition and exercise
- **Different Approaches to Weight Loss**
    - o Diets (e.g., keto, paleo, intermittent fasting)
    - o Exercise routines
    - o Behavioral and psychological strategies
- **Choosing the Right Path for You**
    - o Personalized approaches
    - o Setting realistic goals

CHAPTER 3: NUTRITION AND DIET

- **The Role of Nutrition**
  - o Understanding macronutrients and micronutrients
  - o Importance of balanced eating
- **Creating a Sustainable Diet Plan**
  - o Meal planning and prepping
  - o Healthy recipes and snack ideas
- **Dealing with Cravings and Emotional Eating**
  - o Strategies to manage cravings
  - o Coping mechanisms for emotional eating

CHAPTER 4: EXERCISE AND FITNESS

- **Finding the Right Exercise Routine**
  - o Types of exercise (cardio, strength training, flexibility)
  - o Creating a balanced workout plan
- **Staying Motivated and Consistent**
  - o Setting fitness goals
  - o Tracking progress
- **Overcoming Obstacles**
  - o Common challenges and how to tackle them
  - o Tips for staying on track

CHAPTER 5: MINDSET AND MENTAL HEALTH

- **The Psychological Aspect of Weight Loss**
    - o Importance of mental health in weight loss
    - o Developing a positive mindset
- **Building Self-Esteem and Confidence**
    - o Overcoming negative self-talk
    - o Celebrating small victories
- **Stress Management Techniques**
    - o Mindfulness and meditation
    - o Coping strategies for stress

CHAPTER 6: REAL-LIFE STORIES AND INSPIRATIONS

- **Personal Success Stories**
  - o Interviews with individuals who have succeeded
  - o Lessons learned from their journeys
- **Lessons from Failure**
  - o Understanding setbacks
  - o How to bounce back stronger

CHAPTER 7: MAINTAINING THE WEIGHT LOSS

- **Transitioning to Maintenance Mode**
  - o Adjusting diet and exercise
  - o Long-term strategies for staying fit
- **Staying Accountable**
  - o Tracking your progress
  - o Support systems and communities
- **Preventing Relapse**
  - o Recognizing triggers
  - o Developing a lifelong healthy lifestyle

CHAPTER 8: RESOURCES AND TOOLS

- **Workout Routines**
  - Sample workout schedules
  - Detailed exercise descriptions
- **Additional Resources**
  - List of books, websites, and apps
  - Contact information for support groups and professionals

INTRODUCTION

Personal Background

Thank you for choosing "Call me Fat; a Journey to Weight Loss." My name is Sylvester Matthew, and I'm here to share a very intimate and life-changing experience with you. My weight has always been a source of struggle for me. My physique has been scrutinized from an early age to adulthood, by both me and by others. My mind and self-esteem, in addition to my physical looks, were all shaped by these events. This book is an expression of my struggles, victories, and priceless life lessons discovered during the journey.

Motivation for Writing This Book

The motivation behind writing this book is multifaceted. Firstly, I wanted to provide a source of inspiration and guidance for those who find themselves in a similar situation. I understand the feelings of frustration, hopelessness, and isolation that often accompany the journey of weight loss. By sharing my experience, I want to reassure and uplift everyone who has ever been called "fat" and felt lessened by that term. Furthermore, I intend to challenge societal perceptions about weight and promote a more understanding and observant approach to this common issue.

Purpose of the Book

The purpose of this book is to serve as a comprehensive guide for anyone looking to embark on their own weight loss journey. This is not just a diet or exercise manual; it is a holistic approach to achieving a healthier lifestyle. By combining personal anecdotes with practical advice, scientific explanations, and motivational tips, I aim to provide a well-rounded resource that addresses every aspect of weight loss. Whether you are at the beginning of your journey or seeking to maintain your progress, this book is designed to support and empower you every step of the way.

What to Expect

You may anticipate an open and sincere narrative of my journey throughout this book, along with practical suggestions and techniques you can use to improve your own situation. I'll talk about the highs and lows, triumphs and failures, and the lessons I learned along the journey. My intention is to give you helpful and enlightening guidance that will not only assist you in reaching your weight loss objectives but also cultivate a better, more positive relationship between your body and mind.

Thank you for picking up "Call me Fat; a Journey to Weight Loss." With any luck, my narrative and the knowledge in these pages will encourage you to start on your own path to a better, happier version of yourself.

CHAPTER 1: THE BEGINNING

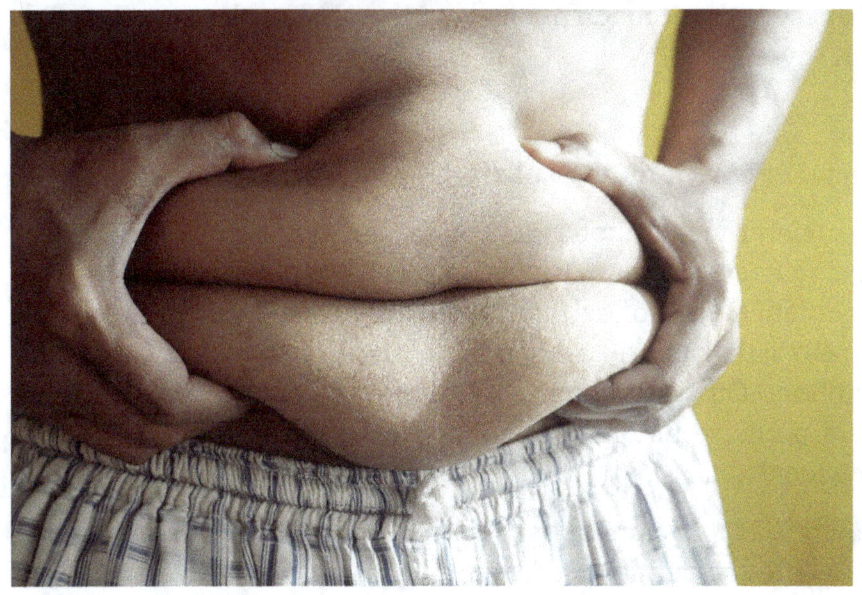

My Struggles with Weight

My weight has influenced my life in a big way ever since I can remember. I was always the overweight child growing up, the one who lagged behind in sports and was made fun of and teased. The school years were particularly difficult for me; although my classmates played with abandon, I was becoming more conscious of my size and the constraints it placed on me. My weight had significant emotional and psychological effects in addition to impairing my physical ability.

As I got older, the difficulties simply got worse. Becoming an adolescent presented new challenges: the need to be attractive, fit in, and have confidence in my own skin. Regretfully, these aspirations frequently seemed unattainable. I detested going shopping for clothes, I got anxious about social situations, and I was always comparing myself to my friends who were slimmer. I was fighting a never-ending internal war; I wanted acceptance—from myself and from other people. Nothing seemed to work long-term, despite my repeated attempts at exercise and nutrition, and every setback made me feel even more hopeless and horrible about myself.

Societal Perceptions and Labels

The societal views about weight, in addition to my own issues, made matters worse. Overweight is generally seen as a sign of indolence, lack of self-control, and even moral failure, while thinness is frequently associated with success, beauty, and self-discipline. Our perceptions of ourselves and how we think others perceive us are shaped by these ubiquitous and sneaky preconceptions.

The label "fat" became a part of my identity, an inescapable tag that seemed to define me entirely. I remember vividly the sting of being called names, the whispering and pointing, the unsolicited advice from strangers about how I should lose weight. These experiences weren't just hurtful; they were dehumanizing. They reinforced the notion that my worth was tied to my physical appearance and that, as a fat person, I was somehow less deserving of respect and kindness.

But the societal perceptions didn't stop there. Media portrayal of overweight individuals further entrenched negative stereotypes. Characters in movies and TV shows often fit a specific mold: the comic relief, the lazy slob, the unattractive sidekick. Rarely were they portrayed as complex, successful, or desirable. This constant bombardment of negative imagery made it even harder to see past my weight and recognize my own value.

Decision to Change

The turning point in my journey came during a particularly low moment. I was at a family gathering, surrounded by loved ones, yet I felt isolated and invisible. The usual comments about my weight resurfaced, well-meaning but ultimately hurtful. As I sat there, listening to the conversations around me, I realized I had two choices: continue on the path of self-destruction and unhappiness or take control of my life and make a change.

Deciding to change wasn't easy. It required a complete shift in mindset and a willingness to confront not just my eating habits and physical activity levels, but also the deep-seated emotional issues tied to my weight. I knew that a superficial approach wouldn't suffice; I needed to address the root causes of my weight gain and develop a sustainable plan for a healthier lifestyle.

I began by educating myself about nutrition and the science of weight loss. I consulted with professionals, including a dietitian and a personal trainer, to develop a personalized plan that would work for me. More importantly, I worked on my mental health, seeking therapy to deal with the emotional scars left by years of bullying and self-criticism. I learned to set realistic goals, celebrate small victories, and be kinder to myself.

The journey was far from easy, and there were many setbacks along the way. However, with each small step forward, I felt a renewed sense of purpose and hope. I started to see changes, not just in my physical appearance, but in my confidence, self-esteem, and overall outlook on life. The decision to change marked the beginning of a transformative journey, one that would teach me the true meaning of resilience, self-love, and empowerment.

I will go into more detail about the particular methods and

techniques that I found useful in the upcoming chapters. In addition to sharing my expertise on fitness, mental health, and nutrition, I'll offer helpful advice for anyone starting a weight reduction journey. By sharing my experience, I want to encourage people to have confidence in themselves and start along the path to a happier, healthier life.

CHAPTER 2: UNDERSTANDING WEIGHT LOSS

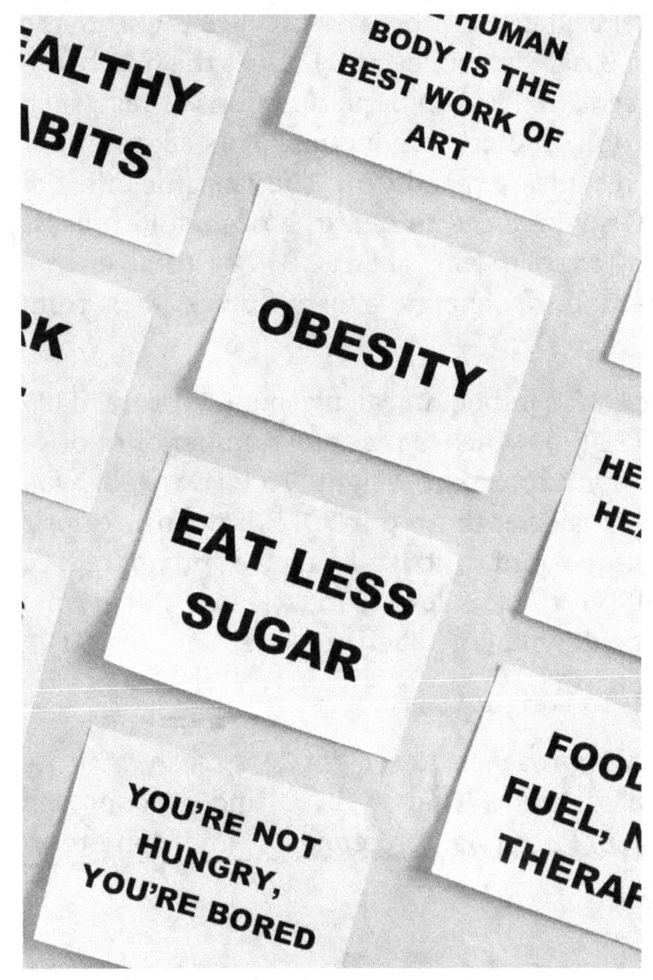

The Science of Weight Loss

It is first necessary to understand the fundamental science guiding weight loss. primarily, when the body burns more calories than it takes in, weight loss happens. We refer to this as generating a deficit in calories. Calories are used by the body for a number of purposes, such as digestion, exercise, and fundamental metabolic activities. The body uses fat reserves as energy when calorie intake is lower than energy expended, which results in weight reduction.

Basics of Metabolism and Calorie Balance

Metabolism refers to the chemical processes that occur within the body to maintain life. Basal Metabolic Rate (BMR) is the number of calories your body needs to perform basic functions at rest, such as breathing, circulation, and cell production. This accounts for about 60-75% of total calorie expenditure. The Thermic Effect of Food (TEF) is the energy required to digest, absorb, and process nutrients from food, contributing about 10% of total energy expenditure. The remaining energy expenditure comes from physical activity and exercise.

Understanding your BMR can help in calculating your total daily energy expenditure (TDEE), which is the total number of calories you need to maintain your current weight. To lose weight, you need to consume fewer calories than your TDEE, creating a caloric deficit. However, it's important to strike a balance and not reduce calories too drastically, as this can lead to muscle loss, nutritional deficiencies, and a slowdown in metabolism.

Different Approaches to Weight Loss

There are numerous approaches to weight loss, each with its own philosophy and methods. The key is to find an approach that aligns with your lifestyle, preferences, and long-term sustainability.

Diets

Various diets can help achieve weight loss, but it's crucial to choose one that is balanced and provides all necessary nutrients.

- **Keto Diet**: A high-fat, low-carb diet that aims to put the body into a state of ketosis, where it burns fat for fuel instead of carbohydrates.
- **Paleo Diet**: Focuses on eating whole foods that our ancestors would have eaten, such as meat, fish, fruits, vegetables, nuts, and seeds, while avoiding processed foods, grains, and dairy.
- **Intermittent Fasting**: Involves cycling between periods of eating and fasting. Common methods include the 16/8 method (fasting for 16 hours and eating during an 8-hour window) and the 5:2 method (eating normally for 5 days and consuming very few calories for 2 non-consecutive days).

Exercise Routines

Exercise is essential for weight loss since it increases the use of calories, promotes muscular growth, and enhances general health.

- **Cardio**: Activities like running, cycling, and swimming that increase heart rate and burn calories. Cardio is effective for burning fat and improving cardiovascular health.
- **Strength Training**: Involves lifting weights or using resistance to build muscle. Muscle tissue burns more calories at rest than fat tissue, so increasing muscle mass can boost metabolism.
- **Flexibility and Balance**: Activities like yoga and Pilates improve flexibility, balance, and overall physical function, complementing other forms of exercise.

Behavioral and Psychological Strategies

Losing weight is a mental as well as physical issue. For long-term success, behavioral and psychological techniques are essential.

- **Mindful Eating**: Overeating can be avoided and a positive relationship with food may be promoted by paying attention to hunger and fullness cues, eating mindfully, and tasting each bite.
- **Behavioral Therapy**: Seeking therapy can assist in addressing psychological obstacles to weight loss, such as emotional eating, body image problems, and others.
- **Support Systems**: Having a support network, consisting of friends, family, or a support group, can offer inspiration, accountability, and support.

Choosing the Right Path for You

Making a decision could be overwhelming due to the abundance of possible approaches. Finding a method that suits your lifestyle and works for you personally is essential.

Personalized Approaches

Everyone's body is different, and what works for one person may not work for another. Consider factors such as your schedule, preferences, and any medical conditions you may have. It may be helpful to consult with healthcare professionals, such as a dietitian, personal trainer, or therapist, to develop a personalized plan.

Setting Realistic Goals

Setting realistic and achievable goals is crucial for maintaining motivation and tracking progress. Start with small, manageable changes and gradually build up to larger goals. Celebrate your achievements along the way, no matter how small they may seem.

Flexibility and Adaptability

Life is unpredictable, and it's important to remain flexible and adaptable in your approach to weight loss. Do not be scared to make changes to your strategy if something isn't working. Identifying an interesting and sustainable approach to a healthy living is the goal.

Long-Term Sustainability

The most effective weight loss plan is one that you can maintain in the long term. Focus on creating long-lasting adjustments to your habits and mindset that support overall health and well-being. Although extreme diets and exercise routines may produce fast results, they are frequently unsustainable and can lead to a vicious cycle of dieting.

Choosing the best approach for you, investigating various strategies, and understanding the science behind weight loss are essential phases in the planning process. We will get more into the details of diet, exercise, and mental health in the upcoming chapters, offering helpful advice and techniques to help you on your journey to a happier, healthier life.

CHAPTER 3: NUTRITION AND DIET

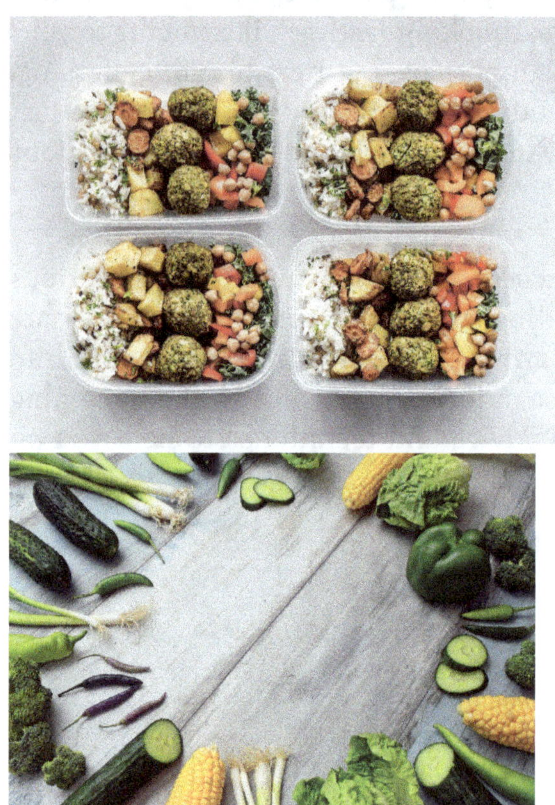

The Role of Nutrition

Nutrition plays a pivotal role in weight loss and overall health. Understanding the basics of nutrition helps you make informed choices about what you eat and how it affects your body.

Understanding Macronutrients and Micronutrients

Macronutrients: These are the nutrients that provide energy and are needed in larger amounts. They include:

- o **Carbohydrates**: The body's primary source of energy. They can be found in fruits, vegetables, grains, and legumes. Aim for complex carbs like whole grains over simple carbs like sugar.
- o **Proteins**: Essential for building and repairing tissues, including muscles. Good sources include meat, fish, dairy, beans, and nuts.
- o **Fats**: Fats are important for energy, cell function, and hormone production. Focus on healthy fats from sources like avocados, nuts, seeds, and olive oil while limiting saturated and trans fats.

Micronutrients: These are vitamins and minerals required in smaller amounts but are crucial for various bodily functions. They include vitamins (such as A, C, D, E, K, and B-complex) and minerals (such as calcium, magnesium, iron, and zinc). Eating a diverse diet rich in fruits, vegetables, lean proteins, and whole grains ensures you get an adequate supply of these nutrients.

Importance of Balanced Eating

A balanced diet provides all the essential nutrients your body needs to function optimally. This means consuming a variety of foods in the right proportions. Here are some key principles:

- **Variety**: Eat a wide range of foods to ensure you get all necessary nutrients.
- **Moderation**: Pay attention to portion sizes to avoid

overeating.

- **Quality**: Choose whole, minimally processed foods over highly processed ones.

Creating a Sustainable Diet Plan

A sustainable diet plan is one that you can stick to in the long term. It should be flexible, enjoyable, and nutritionally balanced.

Meal Planning and Prepping

Meal planning and prepping can save time, reduce stress, and help you make healthier choices. Here's how to get started:

- **Plan Your Meals**: Set aside time each week to plan your meals. Consider your schedule, preferences, and nutritional needs. Aim for balanced meals that include protein, healthy fats, and complex carbohydrates.
- **Create a Shopping List**: Based on your meal plan, make a shopping list to ensure you have all the ingredients you need.
- **Prep in Advance**: Prepare ingredients or whole meals in advance. For example, chop vegetables, cook grains, and portion out snacks. This makes it easier to stick to your plan during busy days.

Healthy Recipes and Snack Ideas

Incorporating a variety of healthy recipes and snacks keeps your diet enjoyable and satisfying. Here are some ideas:

- **Breakfast**: Greek yogurt with berries and nuts, oatmeal with fresh fruit, avocado toast with a poached egg.
- **Lunch**: Quinoa salad with mixed vegetables and grilled chicken, lentil soup with a side of whole-grain bread, tuna salad wrap with whole-wheat tortilla.
- **Dinner**: Baked salmon with roasted vegetables, stir-fry with tofu and brown rice, spaghetti squash with marinara sauce and turkey meatballs.

- **Snacks**: Hummus with carrot sticks, apple slices with almond butter, Greek yogurt with a sprinkle of granola, mixed nuts and seeds.

Dealing with Cravings and Emotional Eating

Cravings and emotional eating can be significant obstacles to maintaining a healthy diet. Understanding and addressing these challenges can help you stay on track.

Strategies to Manage Cravings

Cravings are often driven by emotions, habits, or nutritional deficiencies. Here are some strategies to manage them:

- **Identify Triggers**: Pay attention to what triggers your cravings. Is it stress, boredom, certain environments, or specific foods? Once you identify the triggers, you can develop strategies to manage them.
- **Stay Hydrated**: Sometimes thirst is mistaken for hunger. Drink water throughout the day to stay hydrated.
- **Eat Regularly**: Skipping meals can lead to intense cravings. Eat regular, balanced meals and snacks to keep your blood sugar levels stable.
- **Choose Healthy Alternatives**: Satisfy cravings with healthier options. For example, if you crave something sweet, opt for fruit instead of candy. If you crave something salty, try air-popped popcorn instead of chips.

Coping Mechanisms for Emotional Eating

Emotional eating occurs when you use food to cope with emotions rather than to satisfy physical hunger. Here are some ways to address it:

- **Recognize Emotional Hunger**: Learn to distinguish between physical hunger and emotional hunger. Physical hunger builds gradually, while emotional hunger is sudden and often linked to specific emotions or situations.

- **Find Alternative Coping Strategies**: Develop healthy ways to cope with emotions. This could include exercising, meditating, journaling, talking to a friend, or engaging in a hobby.
- **Practice Mindful Eating**: Be present during meals and pay attention to your body's hunger and fullness cues. Eat slowly, savor each bite, and avoid distractions like TV or smartphones.
- **Seek Support**: If emotional eating is a significant issue, consider seeking support from a therapist or counselor who specializes in eating behaviors.

By understanding the role of nutrition, creating a sustainable diet plan, and managing cravings and emotional eating, you can set yourself up for success on your weight loss journey. In the next chapter, we will explore the importance of exercise and how to find a fitness routine that works for you.

CHAPTER 4: EXERCISE AND FITNESS

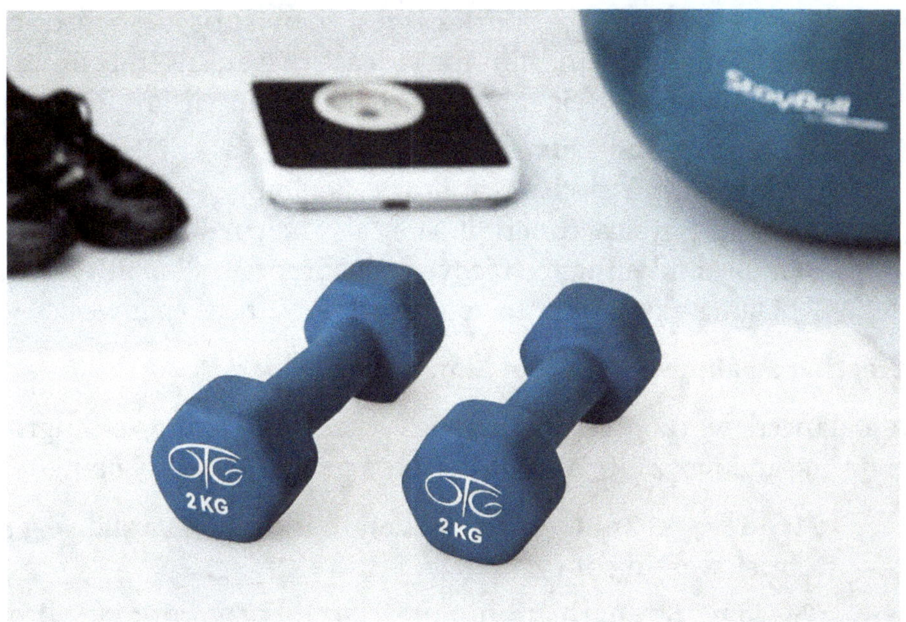

Finding the Right Exercise Routine

One essential element of a good weight loss programme is exercise. It promotes calorie consumption, muscle growth, and general health improvement. Long-term success, however, depends on selecting an exercise programme that fits your personal preferences, way of life, and level of endurance.

Types of Exercise

There are various types of exercises, each offering unique benefits.

Incorporating a mix of these can create a balanced workout plan.

- **Cardio**: Cardiovascular exercises, such as running, cycling, swimming, and dancing, increase heart rate and improve cardiovascular health. They are effective for burning calories and fat. Aim for at least 150 minutes of moderate-intensity or 75 minutes of high-intensity cardio per week.
- **Strength Training**: Strength training, including weight lifting, bodyweight exercises, and resistance band workouts, helps build and maintain muscle mass. Muscle tissue burns more calories at rest than fat tissue, boosting your metabolism. Aim for at least two strength training sessions per week, targeting all major muscle groups.
- **Flexibility and Balance**: Activities like yoga, Pilates, and stretching exercises improve flexibility, balance, and overall physical function. They also help reduce the risk of injury and enhance recovery. Incorporate flexibility and balance exercises into your routine 2-3 times per week.

Creating a Balanced Workout Plan

A balanced workout plan includes a mix of cardio, strength training, and flexibility exercises. Here's a sample weekly plan:

- **Monday**: 30 minutes of moderate-intensity cardio (e.g., brisk walking or cycling)
- **Tuesday**: Strength training (e.g., full-body workout with weights or resistance bands)
- **Wednesday**: Yoga or stretching for 30 minutes
- **Thursday**: 30 minutes of high-intensity cardio (e.g., running or interval training)
- **Friday**: Strength training (e.g., targeting specific muscle groups)
- **Saturday**: 30 minutes of recreational activity (e.g., hiking, dancing, or playing a sport)
- **Sunday**: Rest or gentle stretching

Adjust this plan based on your fitness level, preferences, and schedule. The key is to find activities you enjoy and can commit to regularly.

Staying Motivated and Consistent

Consistency is crucial for seeing results from your exercise routine. Staying motivated can be challenging, but there are several strategies to help you stay on track.

Setting Fitness Goals

Set clear, achievable fitness goals to keep yourself motivated. Goals can be short-term (e.g., completing a 5K run) or long-term (e.g., losing 20 pounds or building muscle). Make sure your goals are Specific, Measurable, Achievable, Relevant, and Time-bound (SMART).

Tracking Progress

Tracking your progress can provide a sense of accomplishment and help you stay motivated. Keep a workout journal or use fitness apps to log your exercises, track your performance, and monitor your progress. Celebrate your achievements, no matter how small they may seem.

Finding Enjoyable Activities

Enjoying your workouts makes it easier to stay consistent. Experiment with different activities to find what you love. Whether it's dancing, hiking, swimming, or playing a sport, finding joy in exercise can transform it from a chore into a rewarding part of your routine.

Creating a Routine

Establishing a regular exercise routine helps make physical activity a habit. Schedule your workouts at the same time each day or week to build consistency. Treat your exercise sessions as non-negotiable appointments with yourself.

Overcoming Obstacles

Challenges and obstacles are inevitable on your fitness journey. Learning how to overcome them can help you stay on track and maintain your progress.

Common Problems and Strategies for Solving Them

- **Lack of Time**: Busy schedules can make it hard to find time for exercise. Overcome this by scheduling shorter, high-intensity workouts or incorporating physical activity into your daily routine (e.g., taking the stairs, walking during lunch breaks).

- **Plateaus**: Hitting a plateau where progress seems to stall is common. Break through plateaus by varying your workouts, increasing intensity, or trying new activities to challenge your body in different ways.

- **Injuries**: Injuries can derail your fitness routine. Prevent injuries by warming up before workouts, using proper form, and listening to your body. If you do get injured, focus on low-impact activities and consult a healthcare professional for guidance.

- **Lack of Motivation**: It is common to have periods of low motivation. To combat this, make new goals, locate a workout partner to hold you accountable, or enroll in fitness programmes or organizations to get encouragement from others.

Tips for Staying on Track

- **Create a Support System**: Surround yourself with supportive friends, family, or workout partners who encourage and motivate you. Join fitness communities or online forums for additional support.

- **Reward Yourself**: Set up a reward system for meeting your fitness goals. Rewards can be non-food-related, such as treating yourself to a new workout outfit, a massage, or a relaxing day off.

- **Stay Flexible**: Life can be unpredictable, and it's important to remain flexible with your routine. If you miss a workout, don't get discouraged. Focus on getting back on track and continuing your journey.

By finding the right exercise routine, staying motivated and consistent, and overcoming obstacles, you can create a sustainable and enjoyable fitness plan that supports your weight loss goals. In the next chapter, we will explore the importance of mindset and mental health in achieving lasting success.

CHAPTER 5: MINDSET AND MENTAL HEALTH

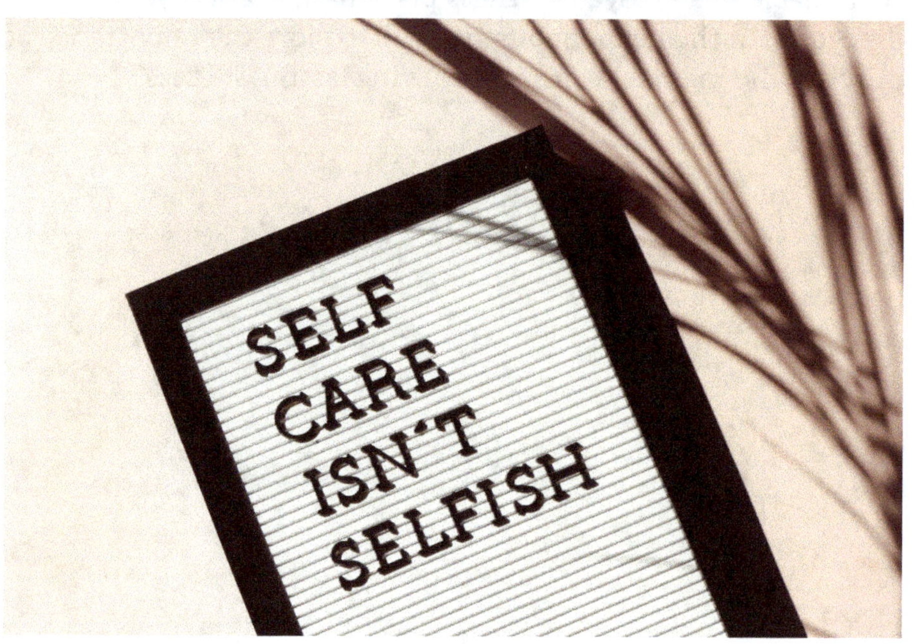

The Psychological Aspect of Weight Loss

Weight loss is not solely a physical endeavor; it is deeply intertwined with your mental and emotional well-being. Understanding the psychological aspects of weight loss can help you address the underlying issues that may hinder your progress and foster a healthier relationship with food, exercise, and your body.

Importance of Mental Health in Weight Loss

Mental health plays a crucial role in weight loss. Emotional states such as stress, anxiety, and depression can significantly impact your eating habits and motivation to exercise. Emotional eating, where food is used as a coping mechanism, can lead to weight gain and hinder weight loss efforts. It's essential to recognize and address these emotional factors to achieve lasting success.

Building a positive mindset towards weight loss involves shifting your focus from simply losing weight to improving your overall health and well-being. This shift can reduce the pressure to achieve a certain number on the scale and encourage more sustainable, healthy behaviors. A positive mindset also helps you bounce back from setbacks and view them as learning opportunities rather than failures.

Building Self-Esteem and Confidence

Low self-esteem and lack of confidence can create significant barriers to weight loss. Building self-esteem and confidence is essential for maintaining motivation and fostering a positive body image.

Overcoming Negative Self-Talk

Negative self-talk, or the critical inner voice that undermines your confidence, can be detrimental to your weight loss journey. Here are some strategies to combat negative self-talk:

- **Awareness**: Recognise patterns in your negative thinking and become conscious of them. You can keep track of these ideas and identify triggers by keeping a journal.
- **Challenge Negative Thoughts**: Question the validity of your negative thoughts and replace them with positive affirmations. For example, instead of thinking, "I'll never lose this weight," tell yourself, "I am making progress every day and becoming healthier."
- **Practice Self-Compassion**: Treat yourself with the same

kindness and understanding you would offer a friend. Acknowledge your efforts and be patient with yourself.

Celebrating Small Victories

Recognizing and celebrating small victories can boost your confidence and motivation. Every step you take towards a healthier lifestyle, no matter how small, is an achievement worth celebrating. Here are some ways to celebrate your progress:

- **Create a Rewards System**: Set milestones and reward yourself when you reach them. Rewards can be non-food-related, such as treating yourself to a new book, a spa day, or a fun activity.

- **Keep a Success Journal**: Write down your achievements, no matter how minor they may seem. Reflecting on your progress can help you stay motivated and appreciate your efforts.

- **Share Your Success**: Share your milestones with supportive friends or family members. Celebrating with others can enhance your sense of accomplishment and provide additional encouragement.

Stress Management Techniques

Stress is a common obstacle in weight loss, as it can lead to emotional eating and disrupt healthy routines. Learning effective stress management techniques can help you maintain your weight loss goals and improve your overall well-being.

Mindfulness and Meditation

Mindfulness and meditation practices can help you manage stress and develop a healthier relationship with food and your body. Here are some techniques to incorporate into your routine:

- **Mindful Eating**: Take note of your meal's flavour, texture, and scent as you enjoy it with your senses. You can identify signs of hunger and fullness and avoid overeating by eating mindfully and slowly, enjoying each bite.

- **Breathing Exercises**: Practice deep breathing exercises to reduce stress and promote relaxation. Try techniques such as diaphragmatic breathing, where you breathe deeply into your abdomen, or the 4-7-8 method, where you inhale for 4 seconds, hold for 7 seconds, and exhale for 8 seconds.

- **Guided Meditation**: Use guided meditation apps or videos to help you relax and focus on the present moment. Regular meditation practice can reduce stress, improve emotional regulation, and enhance overall mental health.

Coping Strategies for Stress

Developing healthy coping strategies for stress can prevent emotional eating and help you stay on track with your weight loss goals. Here are some effective strategies:

- **Physical Activity**: Exercise is a powerful stress reliever. Engage in activities you enjoy, such as walking, dancing, or yoga, to boost your mood and reduce stress levels.

- **Social Support**: Connect with friends, family, or support groups to share your experiences and seek encouragement. Talking to someone who understands your struggles can provide emotional relief and motivation.

- **Hobbies and Interests**: Pursue hobbies and activities that bring you joy and relaxation. Engaging in creative or fulfilling activities can distract you from stress and improve your overall well-being.

- **Time Management**: Organize your schedule to prioritize self-care and avoid feeling overwhelmed. Break tasks into manageable steps, delegate when possible, and set realistic expectations for yourself.

Understanding the psychological aspect of weight loss, building self-esteem and confidence, and managing stress are essential components of a successful weight loss journey. By focusing on your mental and emotional well-being, you can create a positive, sustainable approach to achieving your goals. In the next chapter, we'll delve into real life stories and sources of inspiration to offer encouragement and useful advice from people who have had success with weight loss.

CHAPTER 6: REAL-LIFE STORIES AND INSPIRATIONS

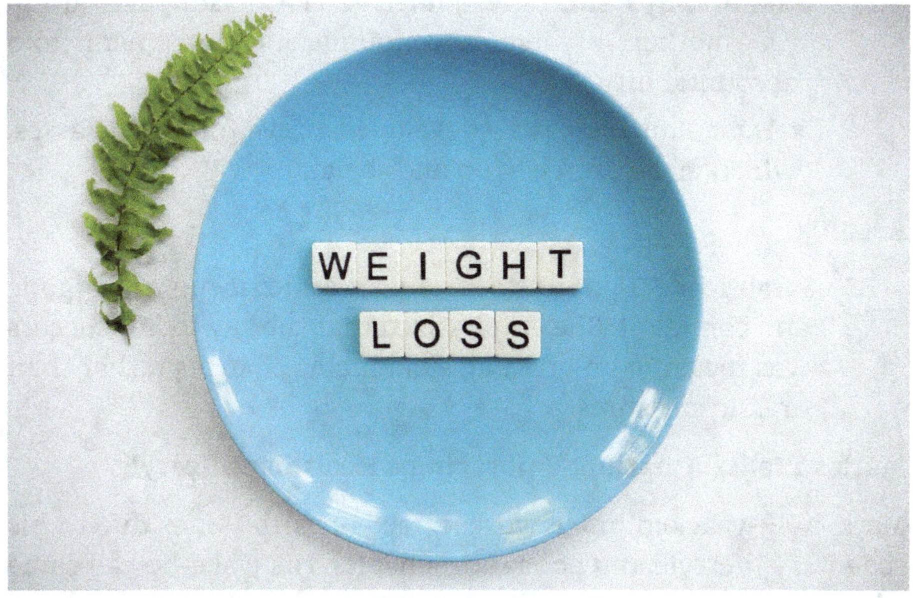

Personal Success Stories

Learning about the successful weight loss achievements of others can be immensely motivational and motivating. These true tales highlight the various routes people have followed to reach their objectives and prove that everyone can succeed with enough willpower and the right approach.

Sarah's Journey: From Struggle to Strength

Sarah, a 35-year-old mother of two, struggled with weight gain after her pregnancies. She found it challenging to balance family responsibilities with self-care. Sarah's turning point came when she realized that taking care of herself was essential for taking care of her family.

Steps Taken:

- **Small Changes**: Sarah started with small, manageable changes. She incorporated more fruits and vegetables into her meals and gradually increased her physical activity by walking with her children.
- **Support System**: She joined a local support group for mothers, where she found encouragement and accountability.
- **Exercise Routine**: Sarah developed a love for Salsa classes, which made exercise fun and social.

Results:

- Sarah lost 50 pounds over a year and felt more energetic and confident. She emphasized that the key to her success was focusing on gradual, sustainable changes rather than drastic measures.

Mark's Transformation: Embracing a Healthier Lifestyle

Mark, a 42-year-old office worker, faced health issues due to his sedentary lifestyle and poor eating habits. His wake-up call came when his doctor warned him about the risks of obesity-related diseases.

Steps Taken:

- **Nutritional Education**: Mark educated himself about nutrition and started meal prepping to avoid unhealthy food choices at work.
- **Fitness Commitment**: He began with simple home workouts and eventually joined a gym. Weight lifting

became his favorite activity.

- **Mindset Shift**: Mark focused on building a positive mindset, celebrating small victories, and not being too hard on himself for occasional setbacks.

Results:

- Mark lost 60 pounds in 18 months and significantly improved his health markers. He now enjoys an active lifestyle and continues to set new fitness goals.

Emily's Path: Overcoming Emotional Eating

Emily, a 29-year-old graduate student, struggled with emotional eating during stressful periods of her studies. She realized that her relationship with food was impacting her physical and mental health.

Steps Taken:

- **Mindful Eating**: Emily practiced mindful eating techniques to recognize true hunger and avoid emotional eating.
- **Therapy and Support**: She sought therapy to address underlying emotional issues and joined an online community of individuals facing similar challenges.
- **Balanced Routine**: Emily incorporated yoga and meditation into her routine, which helped manage stress and improve her overall well-being.

Results:

- Emily lost 40 pounds in a year and developed a healthier relationship with food. She emphasized the importance of addressing emotional health alongside physical health.

Lessons from Failure

Success stories are inspiring, but understanding that failure is part of the journey can be equally valuable. Learning from setbacks and persevering is crucial for long-term success.

John's Struggles: Learning from Setbacks

John, a 50-year-old teacher, experienced several failed attempts at weight loss. He tried multiple diets and exercise plans but found it hard to stick to any of them.

Challenges Faced:

- **Unrealistic Goals**: John often set unrealistic goals, leading to frustration and giving up when results weren't immediate.
- **All-or-Nothing Mentality**: He struggled with an all-or-nothing mindset, where a single slip-up would derail his entire plan.
- **Lack of Support**: John attempted to go through his weight loss journey alone, without seeking support or accountability.

Lessons Learned:

- **Realistic Goals**: John learned to set smaller, achievable goals that kept him motivated and provided a sense of accomplishment.
- **Flexibility**: Embracing flexibility in his approach helped John avoid the all-or-nothing trap. He realized that consistency over perfection was key.
- **Seeking Support**: Finding a supportive community made a significant difference. John joined a local walking group and found online forums where he could share his experiences and receive encouragement.

Lisa's Journey: Overcoming Emotional Barriers

Lisa, a 38-year-old nurse, faced emotional barriers that hindered her weight loss efforts. Stressful work conditions and emotional eating patterns made it difficult for her to maintain a healthy lifestyle.

Challenges Faced:

- **Stress and Burnout**: Lisa's high-stress job led to burnout, which she often coped with by overeating.
- **Negative Self-Talk**: She struggled with negative self-talk and a lack of confidence in her ability to change.
- **Yo-Yo Dieting**: Lisa experienced cycles of extreme dieting followed by weight gain, which affected her physical and emotional health.

Lessons Learned:

- **Self-Compassion**: Lisa learned the importance of self-compassion and treating herself with kindness. She worked on changing her negative self-talk to more positive affirmations.
- **Stress Management**: Developing healthy stress management techniques, such as mindfulness and regular exercise, helped Lisa cope better with her demanding job.
- **Sustainable Changes**: Lisa shifted her focus from quick fixes to sustainable lifestyle changes. She incorporated balanced eating and regular physical activity into her routine.

Conclusion: Embracing Your Unique Journey

Every weight loss journey is unique, with its own set of challenges and triumphs. The stories of Sarah, Mark, Emily, John, and Lisa illustrate that success is possible with determination, the right mindset, and support. Embrace your journey, learn from both successes and setbacks, and remember that every step forward is a step towards a healthier, happier you.

In the next chapter, we will discuss how to maintain your weight loss and develop long-term strategies for staying fit and healthy.

CHAPTER 7: MAINTAINING THE WEIGHT LOSS

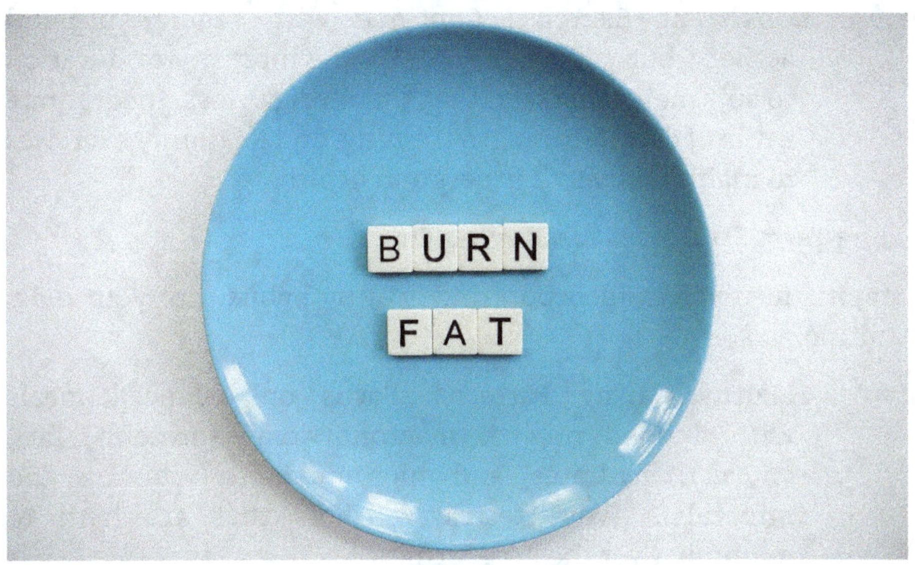

Transitioning to Maintenance Mode

While achieving your weight loss objectives is an important first step, the journey doesn't stop there. Making the switch to maintenance mode is essential to maintaining your results and keeping up your healthy lifestyle.

Adjusting Diet and Exercise

Maintaining weight loss involves finding a balance between your dietary intake and physical activity. Here are some tips for making this transition:

- **Caloric Balance**: As you reach your target weight, you may need to adjust your caloric intake to match your new energy requirements. This typically means eating slightly more than you did during your weight loss phase but still being mindful of portion sizes and overall nutrition.
- **Variety and Flexibility**: Introduce a variety of foods into your diet to ensure you get all necessary nutrients. Being flexible with your eating habits can help prevent boredom and promote long-term adherence.

- **Consistent Exercise**: Continue with regular physical activity, but you might modify the intensity or duration to suit maintenance rather than weight loss. Incorporate a mix of cardio, strength training, and flexibility exercises to maintain overall fitness and health.

Long-term Strategies for Staying Fit

Staying fit involves incorporating healthy habits into your daily routine:

- **Healthy Eating Patterns**: Focus on balanced meals with a good mix of macronutrients (proteins, fats, and carbohydrates) and micronutrients (vitamins and minerals). Avoid restrictive diets that are hard to maintain over the long term.
- **Regular Physical Activity**: Make exercise a non-negotiable part of your lifestyle. Find activities you enjoy and can commit to consistently.
- **Routine Health Checks**: Regularly monitor your weight, body composition, and overall health markers (e.g., blood pressure, cholesterol levels) to ensure you're staying on track.

Staying Accountable

Accountability is key to maintaining your weight loss. It helps you stay focused, motivated, and committed to your new lifestyle.

Tracking Your Progress

Keep track of your progress to stay accountable and identify any potential issues early on:

- **Journaling**: Maintain a food and exercise journal to monitor your daily habits. This can help you recognize patterns and make necessary adjustments.
- **Weigh-ins**: Regular weigh-ins can help you keep track of your weight. However, avoid obsessing over the scale; focus on how you feel and other indicators of health, such as energy levels and clothing fit.
- **Fitness Apps and Devices**: Utilize fitness apps and wearable devices to track your activity levels, calories burned, and other health metrics. These tools can provide insights and keep you motivated.

Support Systems and Communities

Building a support system can provide the encouragement and accountability you need:

- **Family and Friends**: Share your goals and progress with family and friends. Their support can be invaluable.
- **Support Groups**: Join local or online support groups where you can share experiences, gain advice, and find motivation from others on similar journeys.
- **Professional Guidance**: Consider working with a nutritionist, personal trainer, or health coach who can provide personalized advice and support.

Preventing Relapse

Preventing relapse is crucial for long-term success. Recognize potential triggers and develop strategies to manage them effectively.

Recognizing Triggers

Identify situations, emotions, or habits that might lead to weight regain:

- **Stress**: High levels of stress can lead to emotional eating. Recognize stressors in your life and develop healthy coping mechanisms.
- **Social Situations**: Social events often involve food and drink. Plan ahead by deciding what you will eat and drink, and stick to your plan.
- **Habits and Routines**: Certain routines may trigger old habits. Be mindful of these and create new, healthier routines to replace them.

Developing a Lifelong Healthy Lifestyle

Create a sustainable lifestyle that supports your health and weight maintenance:

- **Mindful Eating**: Practice mindful eating by paying attention to hunger and fullness cues. Avoid eating out of boredom, stress, or emotional triggers.
- **Continuous Learning**: Stay informed about nutrition and fitness. As science evolves, so can your approach to maintaining your health.
- **Self-compassion**: Be kind to yourself. Accept that occasional lapses are normal and don't signify failure. Learn from them and move forward.

Conclusion

Maintaining weight loss requires commitment, consistency, and a proactive approach. By transitioning to maintenance mode with a balanced diet and regular exercise, staying accountable through tracking and support systems, and preventing relapse by recognizing triggers and developing a sustainable lifestyle, you can achieve long-term success.

CHAPTER 8: RESOURCES AND TOOLS

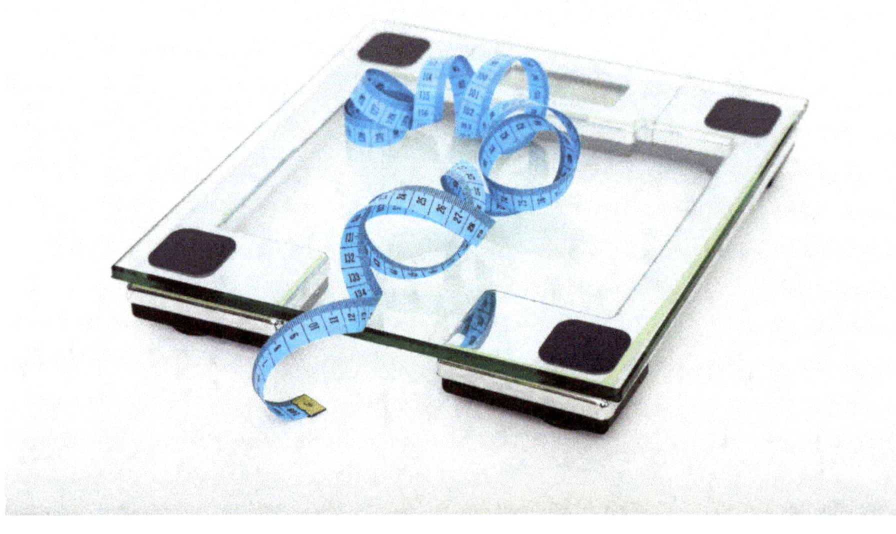

Helpful Apps and Technology

These days, there are a lot of applications and technology tools available that can help you lose weight and keep it off. These programmes can do everything from measure your food consumption and exercise to offer educational materials and motivational support.

Fitness and Nutrition Apps

- **MyFitnessPal**: This popular app allows you to log your meals and track your caloric intake. It has a vast database of foods, making it easy to record what you eat. Additionally, it offers features to log exercise and sync with various fitness devices.

- **Lose It!**: Similar to MyFitnessPal, Lose It! helps you track your food intake and exercise. It provides personalized weight loss plans and has a barcode scanner to quickly input food items.

- **Fitbit**: If you use a Fitbit device, the accompanying app tracks your physical activity, sleep patterns, and even heart rate. It helps set fitness goals and monitor your progress.

- **MyPlate by Livestrong**: This app provides a comprehensive food diary, exercise tracker, and access to a community of users for support and motivation.

- **Headspace**: Mindfulness and meditation are crucial for managing stress and maintaining a positive mindset. Headspace offers guided meditation sessions and mindfulness exercises.

Wearable Technology

- **Fitness Trackers**: Devices like Fitbit, Garmin, and Apple Watch monitor your physical activity, heart rate, and even sleep patterns. These insights can help you stay motivated and on track with your fitness goals.

- **Smart Scales**: Smart scales, such as those from Withings or Fitbit, provide more than just your weight. They can measure body fat percentage, muscle mass, and other health metrics, syncing with your fitness apps for a comprehensive view of your progress.

- **Calorie Counters**: Devices like Jawbone and others offer calorie counting features that can help you track your daily caloric expenditure accurately.

Recommended Reading and Websites

Books and websites can provide in-depth information, inspiration, and support for your weight loss journey. Here are some valuable resources:

Books

- **"The Obesity Code" by Dr. Jason Fung**: This book delves into the science of weight gain and loss, offering insights into how insulin and hormones affect your weight.

- **"Intuitive Eating" by Evelyn Tribole and Elyse Resch**: This book promotes a healthy relationship with food, focusing on listening to your body's hunger and fullness cues rather than following restrictive diets.

- **"Atomic Habits" by James Clear**: While not specifically about weight loss, this book offers practical advice on building and maintaining healthy habits that can be applied to weight loss and fitness.

- **"You Are a Badass" by Jen Sincero**: This motivational book helps boost confidence and encourages a positive mindset, which is crucial for sustaining weight loss.

Websites and Blogs

- **WebMD Weight Loss Clinic**: Provides reliable information on weight loss, nutrition, and fitness, along with tools and tips to help you succeed.

- **Nerd Fitness**: A website and blog that offers a fun, relatable approach to fitness and weight loss, with articles, workouts, and a supportive community.

- **Precision Nutrition**: Offers science-based nutrition and fitness advice, along with articles and guides to help you make informed decisions about your health.

- **Bodybuilding.com**: Not just for bodybuilders, this site provides workout plans, nutrition advice, and a community forum for support and motivation.

Support Groups and Communities

Connecting with others who share similar goals can provide valuable support, motivation, and accountability. Here are some ways to find support:

Online Forums and Communities

- **Reddit**: Subreddits like r/loseit and r/fitness offer a supportive community where you can share your progress, ask for advice, and find inspiration.
- **MyFitnessPal Community**: Engage with other users on the MyFitnessPal forums to share tips, recipes, and motivational stories.
- **SparkPeople**: An online community offering weight loss resources, including forums, blogs, and personalized weight loss plans.

Local Support Groups

- **Weight Watchers**: Offers both online and in-person meetings, providing a structured program and a supportive community to help you reach your weight loss goals.
- **TOPS (Take Off Pounds Sensibly)**: A nonprofit weight loss support organization that offers weekly meetings to provide encouragement and accountability.

- **Meetup**: Search for local fitness and weight loss groups on Meetup.com to find like-minded individuals who can offer support and motivation.

Conclusion

Utilizing these resources and tools can significantly enhance your weight loss journey and help you maintain your progress. From apps and wearable technology to books, websites, and support groups, there are numerous ways to stay informed, motivated, and connected. In the final chapter, we will reflect on the journey, recap key points, and offer encouragement and final thoughts to inspire you to take the first step and continue on your path to a healthier, happier life.

CONCLUSION: CALL ME FAT; A JOURNEY TO WEIGHT LOSS

Reflecting on the Journey

As we reach the conclusion of "Call Me Fat; a Journey to Weight Loss," it's essential to take a moment to reflect on the path we've traveled together. This journey has been about more than just shedding weight; it's been about transforming our lives, embracing our true selves, and discovering the strength and resilience within us.

The Struggles and Triumphs

Throughout this book, we've explored the many facets of weight loss, from understanding the science behind it to delving into the psychological aspects. We've shared real-life stories of individuals who have faced similar struggles, learning from their successes and setbacks. These stories remind us that we are not alone in our journey and that perseverance and determination can lead to incredible transformations.

We've discussed the importance of nutrition and exercise, emphasizing the need for a balanced and sustainable approach. We've learned about the power of mindset and mental health, understanding that a positive outlook and self-compassion are vital components of lasting change. We've also explored practical tools and resources that can support us along the way, from helpful apps and technology to supportive communities and insightful readings.

Celebrating Small Victories

Every step forward, no matter how small, is a victory worth celebrating. Whether it's choosing a healthier meal, completing a workout, or simply being kinder to ourselves, these moments of progress contribute to our overall success. Reflecting on these small victories helps us recognize our growth and keeps us motivated to continue on our path.

Embracing the Journey

Weight loss is not a linear process; it's a journey with ups and downs, challenges and triumphs. Embracing this journey means accepting that setbacks are a natural part of the process and viewing them as opportunities for growth rather than failures. It's about being patient with ourselves and understanding that sustainable change takes time.

Call to Action

Now, as we conclude this book, I want to encourage you to take the next step in your journey. Whether you're just starting or have already made significant progress, remember that every day is an opportunity to move closer to your goals.

Start Today

There's no better time than now to take action. Begin by setting small, achievable goals that align with your long-term vision. Whether it's incorporating more vegetables into your diet, taking a daily walk, or practicing mindfulness, these small steps can lead to significant changes over time.

Seek Support

Reach out to friends, family, or support groups to share your journey and find encouragement. Surround yourself with positive influences who can offer motivation and accountability.

Remember, you don't have to do this alone.

Stay Committed

Commit to yourself and your health. Understand that this journey is about more than just weight loss; it's about improving your overall well-being and quality of life. Stay focused on your goals, celebrate your progress, and be kind to yourself along the way.

Connect with the Author

I'm here to support you on your journey. Feel free to reach out to me through social media or my website. Share your stories, ask questions, and connect with others who are on a similar path. Together, we can inspire and motivate each other to achieve our goals.

Final Thoughts

Weight loss is a deeply personal and transformative journey. It requires dedication, resilience, and a willingness to embrace change. As you move forward, remember that you have the power to create the life you desire. Believe in yourself, stay committed, and never give up.

Thank you for allowing me to be a part of your journey. I hope this book has provided you with the knowledge, tools, and inspiration you need to succeed. Remember, every step you take brings you closer to a healthier, happier you.

Here's to your success and to the incredible journey ahead.

With gratitude and encouragement,

Dr Sylvester Mtthew.

Appendices

Appendix 1: Meal Plans and Recipes

Maintaining a healthy diet is crucial for weight loss and overall well-being. Here are some sample meal plans and recipes to get you started on your journey.

Sample Meal Plans

7-Day Balanced Meal Plan

DAY 1:

- **Breakfast**: Greek yogurt with honey, mixed berries, and a sprinkle of granola
- **Lunch**: Grilled chicken salad with mixed greens, cherry tomatoes, cucumber, and balsamic vinaigrette
- **Snack**: Apple slices with almond butter
- **Dinner**: Baked salmon with quinoa and steamed broccoli

DAY 2:

- **Breakfast**: Overnight oats with chia seeds, banana, and almond milk
- **Lunch**: Quinoa and black bean bowl with avocado, salsa, and lime
- **Snack**: Carrot sticks with hummus
- **Dinner**: Stir-fried tofu with mixed vegetables and brown rice

DAY 3:

- **Breakfast**: Smoothie with spinach, frozen berries, protein powder, and coconut water
- **Lunch**: Turkey wrap with whole grain tortilla, lettuce, tomato, and mustard
- **Snack**: Greek yogurt with honey and walnuts
- **Dinner**: Spaghetti squash with marinara sauce and lean ground turkey

DAY 4:

- **Breakfast**: Scrambled eggs with spinach and whole grain toast
- **Lunch**: Lentil soup with a side of mixed green salad
- **Snack**: Sliced bell peppers with guacamole
- **Dinner**: Grilled shrimp with couscous and roasted Brussels sprouts

DAY 5:

- **Breakfast**: Avocado toast with a poached egg on whole grain bread
- **Lunch**: Chickpea salad with cucumber, cherry tomatoes, red onion, and feta cheese
- **Snack**: Handful of mixed nuts
- **Dinner**: Chicken stir-fry with mixed vegetables and brown rice

DAY 6:

- **Breakfast**: Smoothie bowl with acai, banana, granola, and coconut flakes
- **Lunch**: Tuna salad with mixed greens, olives, and lemon dressing
- **Snack**: Cottage cheese with pineapple
- **Dinner**: Beef and vegetable kebabs with a side of quinoa

DAY 7:

- **Breakfast**: Oatmeal with cinnamon, apple slices, and a drizzle of maple syrup
- **Lunch**: Spinach and mushroom frittata with a side of mixed greens
- **Snack**: Fresh berries and a handful of almonds
- **Dinner**: Grilled chicken with sweet potato and asparagus

Healthy Recipes

Baked Salmon with Quinoa and Steamed Broccoli

Ingredients:

- o 4 salmon filets
- o 1 cup quinoa
- o 2 cups broccoli florets
- o 2 tbsp olive oil
- o 1 lemon (sliced)
- o Salt and pepper to taste

Instructions:

1. Preheat the oven to 375°F (190°C).
2. Place salmon filets on a baking sheet, drizzle with olive oil, and season with salt and pepper. Top with lemon slices.
3. Bake salmon for 20 minutes or until fully cooked.
4. Cook quinoa according to package instructions.
5. Steam broccoli until tender.
6. Serve salmon with quinoa and steamed broccoli on the side.

Overnight Oats with Chia Seeds and Banana.

Ingredients:

o 1/2 cup rolled oats
o 1 tbsp chia seeds
o 1 cup almond milk
o 1 banana (sliced)
o 1 tbsp honey

Instructions:

1. In a mason jar or container, combine oats, chia seeds, and almond milk.
2. Stir well, cover, and refrigerate overnight.
3. In the morning, top with sliced banana and drizzle with honey before serving.

Appendix 2: Workout Routines

Exercise is a key component of weight loss and maintaining a healthy lifestyle. Here are some sample workout routines to help you stay active and fit.

Beginner Workout Routine

Cardio and Strength Training (3 days a week)

DAY 1:

- **Warm-up**: 5 minutes of light jogging or brisk walking
- **Cardio**: 20 minutes of moderate-intensity cardio (e.g., cycling, brisk walking, or elliptical)
- **Strength Training**:
    - Squats: 3 sets of 12 reps
    - Push-ups (modified if needed): 3 sets of 10 reps
    - Dumbbell rows: 3 sets of 12 reps (each arm)
    - Plank: 3 sets of 30 seconds

DAY 2:

- **Warm-up**: 5 minutes of light jogging or brisk walking
- **Cardio**: 20 minutes of interval training (alternating 1 minute of high-intensity with 1 minute of low-intensity)

- **Strength Training**:
    o Lunges: 3 sets of 12 reps (each leg)
    o Shoulder press: 3 sets of 12 reps
    o Bicep curls: 3 sets of 12 reps
    o Russian twists: 3 sets of 20 reps

DAY 3:

- **Warm-up**: 5 minutes of light jogging or brisk walking
- **Cardio**: 20 minutes of steady-state cardio (e.g., jogging, swimming, or rowing)
- **Strength Training**:
  - Deadlifts: 3 sets of 12 reps
  - Tricep dips: 3 sets of 10 reps
  - Side planks: 3 sets of 30 seconds (each side)
  - Bicycle crunches: 3 sets of 20 reps

Intermediate Workout Routine

Cardio and Strength Training (5 days a week)

DAY 1:

- **Warm-up**: 5 minutes of dynamic stretching
- **Cardio**: 30 minutes of running or cycling
- **Strength Training**:
    - o Bench press: 4 sets of 10 reps
    - o Bent-over rows: 4 sets of 10 reps
    - o Squat jumps: 4 sets of 15 reps
    - o Leg raises: 4 sets of 15 reps

DAY 2:

- **Warm-up**: 5 minutes of dynamic stretching
- **Cardio**: 30 minutes of HIIT (high-intensity interval training)
- **Strength Training**:
    o Overhead press: 4 sets of 10 reps
    o Lunges with dumbbells: 4 sets of 12 reps (each leg)
    o Tricep extensions: 4 sets of 12 reps
    o Mountain climbers: 4 sets of 20 reps

DAY 3:

- **Rest or Active Recovery**: Light yoga, stretching, or a leisurely walk

DAY 4:

- **Warm-up**: 5 minutes of dynamic stretching
- **Cardio**: 30 minutes of steady-state cardio (e.g., swimming or rowing)
- **Strength Training**:
  - o Deadlifts: 4 sets of 10 reps
  - o Pull-ups (assisted if needed): 4 sets of 10 reps
  - o Step-ups with dumbbells: 4 sets of 12 reps (each leg)
  - o Flutter kicks: 4 sets of 20 reps

DAY 5:

- **Warm-up**: 5 minutes of dynamic stretching
- **Cardio**: 30 minutes of running or cycling
- **Strength Training**:
  - Incline bench press: 4 sets of 10 reps
  - Dumbbell flyes: 4 sets of 12 reps
  - Goblet squats: 4 sets of 15 reps
  - Plank with shoulder taps: 4 sets of 20 reps

DAY 6:

- **Rest or Active Recovery**: Light yoga, stretching, or a leisurely walk

DAY 7:

- **Warm-up**: 5 minutes of dynamic stretching
- **Cardio**: 30 minutes of HIIT (high-intensity interval training)
- **Strength Training**:
    - o Single-leg deadlifts: 4 sets of 12 reps (each leg)
    - o Dumbbell curls: 4 sets of 12 reps
    - o Tricep dips: 4 sets of 10 reps
    - o Russian twists: 4 sets of 20 reps

Appendix 3: Additional Resources

To further support your weight loss journey, here are some additional resources that can provide valuable information, motivation, and community support.

Books

- **"The Obesity Code" by Dr. Jason Fung**: A deep dive into the science of obesity and strategies for effective weight loss.
- **"Intuitive Eating" by Evelyn Tribole and Elyse Resch**: A guide to developing a healthy relationship with food.
- **"Atomic Habits" by James Clear**: Insights on building and maintaining positive habits.
- **"You Are a Badass" by Jen Sincero**: Motivational book to boost confidence and promote a positive mindset.

Websites and Blogs

- **WebMD Weight Loss Clinic**: Comprehensive information on weight loss, nutrition, and fitness.

- **Nerd Fitness**: Offers articles, workouts, and a supportive community with a fun approach to fitness.
- **Precision Nutrition**: Science-based nutrition and fitness advice with in-depth articles and guides.
- **Bodybuilding.com**: Provides workout plans, nutrition advice, and community support.

Support Groups and Communities

- **Reddit**: Join subreddits like r/loseit and r/fitness for a supportive community.
- **MyFitnessPal Community**: Engage with other users for tips, recipes, and motivational stories.
- **SparkPeople**: An online community offering weight loss resources, including forums and personalized plans.
- **Weight Watchers**: Provides structured programs with online and in-person meetings.
- **TOPS (Take Off Pounds Sensibly)**: Offers weekly meetings for encouragement and accountability.
- **Meetup**: Search for local fitness and weight loss groups to connect with like-minded individuals.

Apps and Technology

- **MyFitnessPal**: Log meals and track caloric intake.
- **Lose It!**: Personalized weight loss plans and food logging.
- **Fitbit**: Tracks physical activity, sleep, and syncs with fitness devices.
- **MyPlate by Livestrong**: Comprehensive food diary and exercise tracker.
- **Headspace**: Offers guided meditation sessions for mindfulness and stress management.

These resources and tools can provide the support and information you need to succeed on your weight loss journey. Remember, the key to lasting change is consistency, patience, and self-compassion. Stay committed, seek support, and celebrate every step forward.